400 Abbreviations & Shorthand
Every RN Should Know

1st Edition

Helen Kim, RN, BSN, CCRN, MPH

400 Abbreviations & Shorthand Every RN Should Know
Text copyright © 2015 by Everyday RN
Image copyright © 2015 by Everyday RN
1st Edition© 2015 by Everyday RN
All rights reserved. Printed in the United States of America.
No part of this book may be used or reproduced in any manner whatsoever
without written permission except in the case of brief quotations embodied
in critical articles and reviews.

Disclaimer
Care has been taken to confirm the accuracy of the information present and
to describe generally accepted practices. However, the author and publisher
are not responsible for errors or omissions or for any consequences from application of the information in this book and make no warranty, expressed
or implied, with respect to the currency, completeness, or accuracy of the
contents of the publication. Application of this information in a particular
situation remains the professional responsibility of the user. Always verify
that abbreviations, methods, and recommendations are congruent with
those set forth by the facility which they are being applied. The names and
situations contained in this book are fictional. References made to trade-
mark products are soley for teaching purposes.

ISBN-13: 978-0986204814
ISBN-10: 0986204811

Contact us at www.everydayrn.com

To Gene, my husband, best friend, and life partner

ABOUT THE AUTHOR

Helen Kim, RN, BSN, CCRN, PHN, MPH, received her bachelor's in Economics and Masters of Public Health from UC Berkeley before going into nursing and received her BSN from the University of Oklahoma Health Sciences Center in 2008. She works in adult critical care, including surgical/trauma ICU and intermediate care/step-down. She also works as a clinical instructor in San Diego where she teaches med-surg and critical care.

ACKNOWLEDGEMENTS

To all the students I have come across, thank you for showing me how you like to learn. I am also grateful for all the nurses and staff I have worked with. I have learned so much from all of you.

CONTENTS

INTRODUCTION

Abbreviations and shorthand are time savers. They will allow you to jam pack a small piece of paper with an incredible amount of information. They also allow you to understand what the heck people in the hospital are talking or writing about. Learning how to survive the medical culture first starts with learning the language. The list below provides widely known abbreviations and shorthand. You may see variations and of course, you will see these abbreviations in both lowercase and uppercase letters. Welcome to the confusing world of medicine!

*Never assume you recognize shorthand or an abbreviation in someone else's notes. Always seek clarification when in doubt.

This book has organized the abbreviations & shorthand in two ways:
1)   The category it makes sense in
2)   Alphabetically

This will allow you to learn words by the category where they make the most sense, and also search the abbreviations with ease. Some abbreviations & shorthand belong in several categories, and therefore have been included more than once.

BY CATEGORY

DEMOGRAPHICS

AND	allow natural death
asp	aspiration
CDiff	clostridium difficile
CPR	cardiopulmonary resuscitation
DNI	do not intubate
DNR	do not resuscitate
DOB	date of birth
DPA	durable power of attorney
DPOA	durable power of attorney
F	female
M	male
MOD	modified
NKA	no known allergies
NKDA	no known drug allergies
PMH	past medical history
POLST	physician's orders for life sustaining treatment
pt	patient
SNF	skilled nursing home
YO	year old

MEDICAL CONDITIONS

ACS	acute coronary syndrome
AICD	automated implantable cardioverter defibrillator
AIDS	acquired immunodeficiency syndrome
AMI	acute myocardial infarction
ARDS	acute respiratory distress syndrome
ARF	acute renal failure
asp	aspiration
AVR	aortic valve replacement/repair
BPH	benign prostatic hypertrophy/hyperplasia
CA	cancer
CABG	coronary artery bypass graft
CAD	coronary artery disease
CAP	community acquired pneumonia
CAPU	community acquired pressure ulcer
CAUTI	community acquired urinary tract infection
CEA	carotid endarterectomy
CHF	congestive heart failure
CLABSI	central line associated blood stream infection
CRE	carbapenem-resistant enterobacteriaceae
COPD	chronic obstructive pulmonary disease
CP	chest pain
cryo	cryoprecipitate

CSF	cerebrospinal fluid
CVA	cerebrovascular accident
DIC	disseminated intravascular coagulation
DM	diabetes mellitus
DT	delirium tremens
DVT	deep vein thrombosis
ESBL	extended spectrum beta-lactamase (resistant organism)
ETOH	alcohol
ex lap	exploratory laparotomy
fem-pop	femoropopliteal bypass
FFP	fresh frozen plasma
Fx	fracture
GERD	gastroesophageal reflux disease
GIB	gastrointestinal bleed
HAI	hospital acquired infection
HAP	hospital acquired pneumonia
HAPU	hospital acquired pressure ulcer
HD	hemodialysis
HIT	heparin-induced thrombocytopenia
HIV	human immunodeficiency virus
HLD	hyperlipidemia
HTN	hypertension
IDDM	insulin-dependent diabetes mellitus
LGIB	lower gastrointestinal bleed
mets	metastasis
MRSA	methicillin-resistant staphylococcus aureus
MVA	motor vehicle accident

MVR	mitral valve replacement/repair
NASH	nonalcoholic steatohepatitis
OA	osteoarthritis
OSA	obstructive sleep apnea
PD	peritoneal dialysis
PE	pulmonary embolism
PFO	patent foramen ovale
PLTs	platelets
PNA	pneumonia
post-op	post-operative
PRBC	packed red blood cells
PU	pressure ulcer
PUD	peptic ulcer disease
RA	rheumatoid arthritis
SAH	subarachnoid hemorrhage
SDH	subdural hematoma
SLE	systemic lupus erythematosus
SOB	shortness of breath
STD	sexually transmitted disease
TB	tuberculosis
TIA	transient ischemic attack
tib-fib fx	tibia fibula fracture
UGIB	upper gastrointestinal bleed
URI	upper respiratory infection
UTI	urinary tract infection
VAP	ventilator associated pneumonia
VRE	vancomycin-resistant enterococci
VTE	venous thromboembolism

NEUROVASCULAR

A&O	alert and oriented
A&Ox3	alert and oriented to person, place, time
A&Ox4	alert and oriented to person, place, time, situation
CSM	circulation, sensation, motion
EENT	ears, eyes, nose, throat
HA	headache
ICP	intracranial pressure
LOC	level of consciousness or loss of consciousness
MCA	middle cerebral artery
PERRL	pupils equal, round, reactive to light
PERRLA	pupils equal, round, reactive to light and accommodation

CARDIOVASCULAR

a-fib	atrial fibrillation
BBB	bundle branch block
BP	blood pressure
CV	cardiovascular
CVP	central venous pressure
EF	ejection fraction
HR	heart rate

IABP	intra-aortic balloon pump
LVEF	left ventricular ejection fraction
MAP	mean arterial pressure
NS	normal sinus
P	pulse
PAC	premature atrial contraction
PEA	pulseless electrical activity
PVC	premature ventricular contraction
RVR	rapid ventricular response
SB	sinus bradycardia
ST	sinus tachycardia
SVT	supraventricular tachycardia
T	temp
V-fib	ventricular fibrillation
VS	vital signs
V-tach	ventricular tachycardia

PULMONARY

AC	assist control
BIPAP	bilevel positive airway pressure
CPAP	continuous positive airway pressure
CPT	chest physiotherapy
CTA	clear to auscultation
EPAP	expiratory positive airway pressure
ET	endotracheal
ETT	endotracheal tube
IPAP	inspiratory positive airway pressure

IPPB	intermittent positive-pressure breathing
IS	incentive spirometry
LLL	left lower lobe
LUL	left upper lobe
O2 sat	oxygen saturation
O2	oxygen
PA	pulmonary artery
PEEP	peak inspiratory end pressure
PFT	pulmonary function test
PIP	peak inspiratory pressure
pulm	pulmonary
resp	respiratory
RLL	right lower lobe
RR	respiratory rate
RUL	right upper lobe
SOB	short of breath
sxn	suction
trach	tracheostomy
TV	tidal volume
V/Q	ventilation/perfusion
vent	ventilator

GASTROINTESTIONAL

BG	blood glucose
BM	bowel movement
BS	bowel sounds

BS	blood sugar
GI	gastrointestinal
LBM	last bowel movement
LLQ	left lower quadrant
LUQ	left upper quadrant
N/V	nausea vomiting
NG	nasogastric
PEG or G-tube	percutaneous endoscopic gastrostomy
PEJ or J-tube	percutaneous endoscopic jejunostomy
PPN	peripheral parenteral nutrition
RLQ	right lower quadrant
RUQ	right upper quadrant
TPN	total parenteral nutrition

GENITOURINARY

GU	genitourinary
HD	hemodialysis
I&O	intake and output
neph	nephrostomy
PD	peritoneal dialysis
UOP	urine output

SKIN

CAPU	community acquired pressure ulcer
dsg	dressing
HAPU	hospital acquired pressure ulcer
PU	pressure ulcer
VSU	venous stasis ulcer

ACTIVITY/MOBILITY

ad lib	at liberty
ADL	activities of daily living
BLE	bilateral lower extremities
BRP	bathroom privileges
BUE	bilateral upper extremities
C-spine	cervical spine
HOB	head of bed
LLE	left lower extremity
LUE	left upper extremity
OOB	out of bed
RLE	right lower extremity
ROM	range of motion
RUE	right upper extremity
xfr	transfer

LINES

AC	antecubital
a-line	arterial line
CT	chest tube
CVC	central venous catheter
CVP	central venous pressure
F	foley
FT	feeding tube
G	gauge
IJ	internal jugular
LCS	low continuous suction
NG	nasogastric
NGT	nasogastric tube
OG	orogastric
PICC	peripherally inserted central catheter
PIV	peripheral intravenous catheter
TF	tube feeding

DRIPS/MEDICATIONS

abx	antibiotics
amio	amiodarone
ASA	aspirin
BB	beta-blocker

BDZ	benzodiazepines
CCB	calcium channel blocker
D10/D10W	dextrose 10%
D5/D5W	dextrose 5%
dig	digoxin
dilt	diltiazem
dopa	dopamine
epi	epinephrine
ER	extended-release
gent	gentamycin
gtt	drip
H2O2	hydrogen peroxide
hep	heparin
IR	immediate-release
IVF	IV fluids
KCL	potassium chloride
KVO	keep vein open
levo	levophed
meds	medications
MIV	maintenance intravenous fluids
MOM	milk of magnesia
MS	morphine sulphate
NaCl	sodium chloride
neo	neosynephrine
NS	normal saline
NSAID	nonsteroidal anti-inflammatory drug
ntg	nitroglycerine
oxy	oxycodone
PCN	penicillin
PPI	proton pump inhibitor

Rx	prescription, drug, pharmacy
SR	sustained-release
SSRI	selective serotonin reuptake inhibitor
tPA	tissue plasminogen activator
TPN	total parenteral nutrition
vanco	vancomycin
vitK	vitamin K

LABS/MICROBIOLOGY

ABG	arterial blood gas
AFB	acid-fast bacilli
aPTT	activated partial thromboplastin time
BC	blood culture
BMP	basic metabolic panel
Ca	calcium
CBC	complete blood count
CI	cardiac index
Cl	chloride
CMP	complete metabolic panel
CO	cardiac output
CO_2	carbon dioxide
H&H	hemoglobin & hematocrit
Hct	hematocrit
Hgb	hemoglobin
INR	international normalized ratio
K	potassium
LP	lumbar puncture

lytes	electrolytes
Mg	magnesium
micro	microbiology
Na	sodium
Plts	platelets
PTT	partial thromboplastin time
RBC	red blood cell
Svo2	percentage of oxygen saturation in the pulmonary arterial blood
UA	urinalysis
UC	urine culture
WBC	white blood count

DIAGNOSTICS/PROCEDURES

angio	angiogram
CAT	computerized axial tomography (same as CT)
CT	computerized tomography
CXR	chest x-ray
D&C	dilation & curettage
ECG/EKG	electrocardiogram
ECHO	echocardiogram
EEG	electroencephalogram
EGD	esophagogastroduodenoscopy
HIDA scan	hepatobiliary iminodiacetic acid scan
KUB	kidney ureter bladder x-ray
LP	lumbar puncture

MIBI	methoxyisobutylisonitrile (used in MIBI stress test)
MRI	magnetic resonance imaging
nuc med	nuclear medicine
PCI	percutaneous coronary intervention
PCTA	percutaneous transluminal coronary angioplasty
PET	positron imaging tomography
US	ultrasound
XR	x-ray

MISCELLANEOUS

+	positive
-	negative
2°	secondary to
Δ	change
Ø	none
@	at
AC	before meals
AC/HS	before meals and before bedtime
ASAP	as soon as possible
BID	twice daily
BPM	beats per minute
BSA	body surface area
cm	centimeter
c/o	complains of
DC	discharge, discontinue

Dx	diagnosis
Fr	french
F/U	follow-up
fxn	function
g	gram
H/O	history of
HS	before bedtime
Hx	history
ICD	intermittent compression device
IM	intramuscular
in	inch
IV	intravenous
IVP	IV push
IVPB	IV piggy-back
kg	kilogram
L	left
L	liter
lb	pound
mcg	microgram
mEq	milliequivalents
mg	milligram
mL	milliliter
mmHg	millimeters of mercury
NPO	nothing by mouth
PC	after meals
po	by mouth
POD	post-op day
PRN	as needed
q	every
QAM	every morning

QID	four times daily
QPM	every evening
R	right
SCD	sequential compression device
s/p	status post
SQ	subcutaneous
STAT	immediately
TID	three times daily
Tx	treatment
w/	with
WDL	within defined limits
WNL	within normal limits
wt	weight
x	times (referring to number of times)

HEALTH CARE WORKERS

APRN	advanced practice registered nurse
cardio	cardiologist
CNS	clinical nurse specialist
COD	cardiologist on duty
DO	doctor of osteopathy
GS	general surgery
LCSW	licensed clinical social worker
LPN	licensed practical nurse
MA	medical assistant
MD	medical doctor
MOD	medical (doctor) on duty

neph	nephrologist
Ob/Gyn	obstetrics and gynecology
OT	occupational therapy/therapist
PA	physician's assistant
peds	pediatrics
PharmD	doctor of pharmacy
PT	physical therapy/therapist
RD	registered dietitian
RN	registered nurse
RPh	registered pharmacist
RT	respiratory therapist
SOD	surgeon on duty
uro	urologist

HOSPITAL DEPARTMENTS

cath lab	cardiac catheterization lab
CCU	coronary care unit
DOU	definitive observation unit
ED	emergency department
ER	emergency room (same as ED)
heme/onc	hematology/oncology
ICU	intensive care unit
IMU	intermediate care unit
IR	interventional radiology
M/S	medical-surgical (non-telemetry)
med-surg	medical-surgical (non-telemetry)
MICU	medical intensive care unit

NICU	neonatal intensive care unit
OR	operating room
PACU	post-anesthesia care unit
PCU	progressive care unit
PICU	pediatric intensive care unit
SICU	surgical intensive care unit
tele	telemetry
TICU	trauma intensive care unit

ALPHABETICAL LIST

ALPHABETICAL LIST

-	negative
@	at
Δ	none
+	positive
Ø	change
2°	secondary to
a-fib	atrial fibrillation
a-line	arterial line
A&O	alert and oriented
A&Ox3	alert and oriented to person, place, time
A&Ox4	alert and oriented to person, place, time, situation
ABG	arterial blood gas
abx	antibiotics
AC	antecubital
AC	assist control
AC	before meals
AC/HS	before meals and before bedtime
ACS	acute coronary syndrome
ad lib	at liberty
ADL	activities of daily living

AFB	acid-fast bacilli
AICD	automated implantable cardioverter defibrillator
AIDS	acquired immunodeficiency syndrome
AMI	acute myocardial infarction
amio	amiodarone
AND	allow natural death
angio	angiogram
APRN	advanced practice registered nurse
aPTT	activated partial thromboplastin time
ARDS	acute respiratory distress syndrome
ARF	acute renal failure
ASA	aspirin
ASAP	as soon as possible
asp	aspiration
AVR	aortic valve replacement/repair
BB	beta-blocker
BBB	bundle branch block
BC	blood culture
BDZ	benzodiazepines
BG	blood glucose
BID	twice daily
BIPAP	bilevel positive airway pressure
BLE	bilateral lower extremities
BM	bowel movement
BMP	basic metabolic panel
BP	blood pressure
BPH	benign prostatic hypertrophy/hyperplasia
BPM	beats per minute
BRP	bathroom privileges

BS	blood sugar or bowel sounds
BSA	body surface area
BUE	bilateral upper extremities
C-spine	cervical spine
c/o	complains of
Ca	calcium
CA	cancer
CABG	coronary artery bypass graft
CAD	coronary artery disease
CAP	community acquired pneumonia
CAPU	community acquired pressure ulcer
cardio	cardiologist
CAT	computerized axial tomography (same as CT)
cath lab	cardiac catheterization lab
CAUTI	community acquired urinary tract infection
CBC	complete blood count
CCB	calcium channel blocker
CCU	coronary care unit
CDiff	clostridium difficile
CEA	carotid endarterectomy
CHF	congestive heart failure
CI	cardiac index
Cl	chloride
CLABSI	central-line associated bloodstream infection
cm	centimeter
CMP	complete metabolic panel
CNS	clinical nurse specialist
CO	cardiac output

CO_2	carbon dioxide
COD	cardiologist on duty
COPD	chronic obstructive pulmonary disease
CP	chest pain
CPAP	continuous positive airway pressure
CPR	cardiopulmonary resuscitation
CPT	chest physiotherapy
CRE	carbapenem-resistant enterobacteriaceae
cryo	cryoprecipitate
CSF	cerebrospinal fluid
CSM	circulation, sensation, motion
CT	chest tube
CT	computerized tomography
CTA	clear to auscultation
CV	cardiovascular
CVA	cerebrovascular accident
CVC	central venous catheter
CVP	central venous pressure
CXR	chest x-ray
D&C	dilation & curettage
D10/D10W	dextrose 10%
D5/D5W	dextrose 5%
DC	discharge, discontinue
DIC	disseminated intravascular coagulation
dig	digoxin
dilt	diltiazem
DM	diabetes mellitus
DNI	do not intubate
DNR	do not resuscitate
DO	doctor of osteopathy

DOB	date of birth
dopa	dopamine
DOU	definitive observation unit
DPOA/DPA	durable power of attorney
dsg	dressing
DT	delirium tremens
DVT	deep vein thrombosis
Dx	diagnosis
ECG/EKG	electrocardiogram
ECHO	echocardiogram
ED	emergency department
EEG	electroencephalogram
EENT	ears, eyes, nose, throat
EF	ejection fraction
EGD	esophagogastroduodenoscopy
EPAP	expiratory positive airway pressure
epi	epinephrine
ER	emergency room (same as ED)
ER	extended-release
ESBL	extended spectrum beta-lactamase (resistant organism)
ET	endotracheal
ETOH	alcohol
ETT	endotracheal tube
ex lap	exploratory laparotomy
F	female
F/U	follow-up
fem-pop	femoropopliteal bypass
FFP	fresh frozen plasma
Fr	french

FT	feeding tube
Fx	fracture
fxn	function
G	gauge
g	gram
gent	gentamycin
GERD	gastroesophageal reflux disease
GI	gastrointestinal
GIB	gastrointestinal bleed
GS	general surgery
gtt	drip
GU	genitourinary
H&H	hemoglobin & hematocrit
H/O	history of
H2O2	hydrogen peroxide
HA	headache
HAI	hospital acquired infection
HAP	hospital acquired pneumonia
HAPU	hospital acquired pressure ulcer
Hct	hematocrit
HD	hemodialysis
heme/onc	hematology/oncology
hep	heparin
Hgb	hemoglobin
HIDA scan	hepatobiliary iminodiacetic acid scan
HIT	heparin-induced thrombocytopenia
HIV	human immunodeficiency virus
HLD	hyperlipidemia
HOB	head of bed
HR	heart rate

HS	before bedtime
HTN	hypertension
Hx	history
I&O	intake and output
IABP	intra-aortic balloon pump
ICD	intermittent compression device
ICP	intracranial pressure
ICU	intensive care unit
IDDM	insulin-dependent diabetes mellitus
IJ	internal jugular
IM	intramuscular
IMU	intermediate care unit
in	inch
INR	international normalized ratio
IPAP	inspiratory positive airway pressure
IPPB	intermittent positive-pressure breathing
IR	immediate-release
IR	interventional radiology
IS	incentive spirometry
IV	intravenous
IVF	IV fluids
IVP	IV push
IVPB	IV piggy-back
K	potassium
KCL	potassium chloride
kg	kilogram
KUB	kidney ureter bladder x-ray
KVO	keep vein open
L	left
L	liter

lb	pound
LBM	last bowel movement
LCS	low continuous suction
LCSW	licensed clinical social worker
levo	levophed
LGIB	lower gastrointestinal bleed
LLE	left lower extremity
LLL	left lower lobe
LLQ	left lower quadrant
LOC	level of consciousness or loss of consciousness
LP	lumbar puncture
LP	lumbar puncture
LPN	licensed practical nurse
LUE	left upper extremity
LUL	left upper lobe
LUQ	left upper quadrant
LVEF	left ventricular ejection fraction
lytes	electrolytes
M	male
M/S	medical-surgical (non-telemetry)
MA	medical assistant
MAP	mean arterial pressure
MCA	middle cerebral artery
mcg	microgram
MD	medical doctor
med-surg	medical-surgical (non-telemetry)
meds	medications
mEq	milliequivalents
mets	metastasis

Mg	magnesium
mg	milligram
MIBI	methoxyisobutylisonitrile (used in MIBI stress test)
micro	microbiology
MICU	medical intensive care unit
MIV	maintenance intravenous fluids
mL	milliliter
mmHg	millimeters of mercury
MOD	medical (doctor) on duty
mod	modified
MOM	milk of magnesia
MRI	magnetic resonance imaging
MRSA	methicillin-resistant staphylococcus aureus
MS	morphine sulphate
MVA	motor vehicle accident
MVR	mitral valve replacement/repair
N/V	nausea vomiting
Na	sodium
NaCl	sodium chloride
NASH	nonalcoholic steatohepatitis
neo	neosynephrine
neph	nephrologist
neph	nephrostomy
NG	nasogastric
NG	nasogastric
NGT	nasogastric tube
NICU	neonatal intensive care unit
NKA	no known allergies
NKDA	no known drug allergies

NPO	nothing by mouth
NS	normal saline
NS	normal sinus
NSAID	nonsteroidal anti-inflammatory drug
ntg	nitroglycerine
nuc med	nuclear medicine
O_2	oxygen
O_2 sat	oxygen saturation
OA	osteoarthritis
Ob/Gyn	obstetrics and gynecology
OG	orogastric
OOB	out of bed
OR	operating room
OSA	obstructive sleep apnea
OT	occupational therapy/therapist
oxy	oxycodone
P	pulse
PA	physician's assistant
PA	pulmonary artery
PAC	premature atrial contraction
PACU	post-anesthesia care unit
PC	after meals
PCI	percutaneous coronary intervention
PCN	penicillin
PCTA	percutaneous transluminal coronary angioplasty
PCU	progressive care unit
PD	peritoneal dialysis
PE	pulmonary embolism
PEA	pulseless electrical activity

peds	pediatrics
PEEP	peak inspiratory end pressure
PEG or G-tube	percutaneous endoscopic gastrostomy
PEJ or J-tube	percutaneous endoscopic jejunostomy
PERRL	pupils equal, round, reactive to light
PERRLA	pupils equal, round, reactive to light and accommodation
PET	positron imaging tomography
PFO	patent foramen ovale
PFT	pulmonary function test
PharmD	doctor of pharmacy
PICC	peripherally inserted central catheter
PICU	pediatric intensive care unit
PIP	peak inspiratory pressure
PIV	peripheral intravenous catheter
PLTs	platelets
Plts	platelets
PMH	past medical history
PNA	pneumonia
po	by mouth
POD	post-op day
POLST	physician's orders for life sustaining treatment
post-op	post-operative
PPI	proton pump inhibitor
PPN	peripheral parenteral nutrition
PRBC	packed red blood cells
PRN	as needed
pt	patient
PT	physical therapy/therapist

PTT	partial thromboplastin time
PU	pressure ulcer
PU	pressure ulcer
PUD	peptic ulcer disease
pulm	pulmonary
PVC	premature ventricular contraction
q	every
QAM	every morning
QID	four times daily
QPM	every evening
R	right
RA	rheumatoid arthritis
RBC	red blood cell
RD	registered dietitian
resp	respiratory
RLE	right lower extremity
RLL	right lower lobe
RLQ	right lower quadrant
RN	registered nurse
ROM	range of motion
RPh	registered pharmacist
RR	respiratory rate
RT	respiratory therapist
RUE	right upper extremity
RUL	right upper lobe
RUQ	right upper quadrant
RVR	rapid ventricular response
Rx	prescription, drug, pharmacy
s/p	status post
SAH	subarachnoid hemorrhage

SB	sinus bradycardia
SCD	sequential compression device
SDH	subdural hematoma
SICU	surgical intensive care unit
SLE	systemic lupus erythematosus
SNF	skilled nursing home
SOB	shortness of breath
SOD	surgeon on duty
SQ	subcutaneous
SR	sustained-release
SSRI	selective serotonin reuptake inhibitor
ST	sinus tachycardia
STAT	immediately
STD	sexually transmitted disease
Svo2	percentage of oxygen saturation in the pulmonary arterial blood
SVT	supraventricular tachycardia
sxn	suction
T	temp
TB	tuberculosis
tele	telemetry
TF	tube feeding
TIA	transient ischemic attack
tib-fib fx	tibia fibula fracture
TICU	trauma intensive care unit
TID	three times daily
TKO	to keep open
tPA	tissue plasminogen activator
TPN	total parenteral nutrition
trach	tracheostomy

TV	tidal volume
Tx	treatment
UA	urinalysis
UC	urine culture
UGIB	upper gastrointestinal bleed
UOP	urine output
URI	upper respiratory infection
uro	urologist
US	ultrasound
UTI	urinary tract infection
V-fib	ventricular fibrillation
V-tach	ventricular tachycardia
V/Q	ventilation/perfusion
vanco	vancomycin
VAP	ventilator associated pneumonia
vent	ventilator
vitK	vitamin K
VRE	vancomycin-resistant enterococci
VS	vital signs
VSU	venous stasis ulcer
VTE	venous thromboembolism
w/	with
WBC	white blood count
WDL	within defined limits
WNL	within normal limits
wt	weight
x	times (number of times)
xfr	transfer
XR	x-ray
YO	year old

CONCLUSION

Congratulations! You are one step closer to understanding the ever-confusing nursing language. Learning anything new takes time, but this book saves you countless hours by only giving you the most used and most relevant abbreviations and shorthand you will find in the hospital today. Commit to learning the abbreviations and shorthand in this book and you will truly see a difference in how much you understand at work.

Check out www.everydayRN.com for more useful nursing resources.

Made in the USA
Middletown, DE
23 August 2020